W9-AAC-703

Management Guidelines for Adult Nurse Practitioners

Introducing the NEW
Taber's Cyclopedic Medical Dictionary CD-ROM Multimedia

Taber's Cyclopedic Medical Dictionary CD-ROM Multimedia is just the ticket to meet your need for fast, reliable health science information. Taber's stellar attractions - the most terms (approximately 55,000!), portability, input from expert consultants, and the most comprehensive appendices - are now enhanced with the addition of LIGHTS! CAMERA! ACTION!
... *AND SOUND!*

Also available packaged with the Taber's Dictionary* for only $59.95!

Taber's on CD-ROM has it all!

✓ *Powerful search engine*

✓ *Useful hypertext links*

✓ *Bookmark feature*

✓ *Copy-and-paste*

✓ *Zoom-and-pan viewing*

✓ *Audio pronunciations*

✓ *Videos*

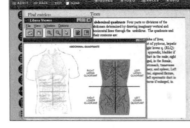

* The Taber's Dictionary/CD-ROM package includes Taber's Cyclopedic Medical Dictionary, 18th Edition (Indexed Version), and Taber's Cyclopedic Medical Dictionary CD-ROM Multimedia

Enhance your professional library with the most comprehensive nursing and health professions dictionary now available on CD-ROM. Order your copy of **Taber's Cyclopedic Medical Dictionary CD-ROM Multimedia** today!

Phone: 800-323-3555   Fax: 215-440-3016

E-mail to: orders@fadavis.com

Also, visit our Home Page at www.fadavis.com

Also available at your local health science bookstore.

Minimum system requirements

For WIN: 386/33 or better; Windows 3.1 or later; 3 MB of hard drive space; 8 MB of RAM; SVGA color monitor; 2X CD-ROM; 8 bit audio (sound card required).

For MAC: 68030 processor (Power PC recommended); Mac OS 7.0 or later; 8 MB RAM; 3 MB hard drive space; 2X CD-ROM; 8 bit audio (sound card required).

0337-1: Taber's Dictionary/CD-ROM Package $59.95.

0306-1: Taber's Cyclopedic Medical Dictionary CD-ROM Multimedia $44.95.

Call for network pricing.

0193-X: Taber's Cyclopedic Medical Dictionary, 18th Ed. Thumb Indexed. $32.95.

0194-8: Taber's Cyclopedic Medical Dictionary, 18th Ed. Plain. $29.95.

Prices are subject to change without notice.

F. A. Davis Company

1915 Arch Street • Philadelphia, PA 19103
215-440-3001 • 1-800-323-3555

MANAGEMENT GUIDELINES FOR ADULT NURSE PRACTITIONERS

Lynne M. Hektor Dunphy, PhD, RN, FNP, CS
Associate Professor, College of Nursing
Florida Atlantic University
Boca Raton, Florida
Adjunct Nurse Researcher
Miami Veterans Administration Medical
  Center
Miami, Florida

 F. A. DAVIS COMPANY • Philadelphia

F. A. Davis Company
1915 Arch Street
Philadelphia, PA 19103

Copyright © 1999 by F. A. Davis Company

All rights reserved. This book is protected by copyright. No part of it may be reproduced, stored in a retrieval system, or transmitted in any form or by any means, electronic, mechanical, photocopying, recording, or otherwise, without written permission from the publisher.

Printed in the United States of America

Last digit indicates print number: 10 9 8 7 6 5 4 3 2 1

Acquisitions Editor: Joanne P. DaCunha, RN, MSN
Production Editor: Michael Schnee
Cover Designer: Louis J. Forgione

As new scientific information becomes available through basic and clinical research, recommended treatments and drug therapies undergo changes. The author(s) and publisher have done everything possible to make this book accurate, up to date, and in accord with accepted standards at the time of publication. The authors, editors, and publisher are not responsible for errors or omissions or for consequences from application of the book, and make no warranty, expressed or implied, in regard to the contents of the book. Any practice described in this book should be applied by the reader in accordance with professional standards of care used in regard to the unique circumstances that may apply in each situation. The reader is advised always to check product information (package inserts) for changes and new information regarding dose and contraindications before administering any drug. Caution is especially urged when using new or infrequenctly ordered drugs.

Library of Congress Cataloging-in-Publication Data

Management guidelines for adult nurse practitioners / [edited by]
   Lynne M. Hektor Dunphy.
       p. cm.
   Includes bibliographical references and index.
   ISBN 0-8036-0229-4 (alk. paper)
   1. Primary care (Medicine)   2. Nurse practitioners.   3. Medical
protocols.   I. Hektor Dunphy, Lynne M.
   [DNLM: 1. Nursing Care.   2. Nursing Assessment. WY 100 M265
1998]
RT82.8.M33 1998
610.73—dc21
DNLM/DLC
for Library of Congress   98-11268
                                                                CIP

Authorization to photocopy items for internal or personal use, or the internal or personal use of specific clients, is granted by F. A. Davis Company for users registered with the Copyright Clearance Center (CCC) Transactional Reporting Service, provided that the fee of $.10 per copy is paid directly to CCC, 222 Rosewood Drive, Salem, MA 01923. For those organizations that have been granted a photocopy licience by CCC, a separate system of payment has been arranged. The fee code for users of the Transactional Reporting Service is: 8036-0229 / 99 0 + $.10.

To my family, especially my husband, Jim,
for his patience and support;
my mother for her encouragement;
and my nieces, Andrea and Autumn, for their love.
Lastly, to my departed father
for his guidance, his understanding,
and, most of all, the memories.

PREFACE

Management Guidelines for Adult Nurse Practitioners is designed for advanced practice nurses and students who are providing primary care to adults. These guidelines were developed by many experts to provide fast and easy access to a variety of types of information needed to manage the care of the adult patient in the primary-care setting. This information will also be useful to physician assistants and physicians in primary care, clinical nurse specialists, case managers, community health nurses, school nurses, and RNs providing ambulatory care and home health care.

Unit I, "The Healthy Adult," reviews information necessary to provide holistic care. Chapter 1, "Growth and Development: Health across the Life Span," reviews important growth and deveopmental content; Chapter 2, "Health Promotion," discusses principles necessary for incorporating health promotion in your practice; and Chapter 3, "Nutrition," summrizes content essential to understanding nutritional principles and their application. This important nursing base is essential to developing your plan of care.

Unit II, "Assessment," reviews important information related to history taking and physical exam. Chapter 4, "History Taking," discusses concrete ways of creating an environment conducive to information gathering and dealing with patients from a variety of cultural backgrounds, including those with language differences. Chapter 5, "Physical Examination and Clinical Decision Making," reviews the important components of the physical exam and diagnostic test data, and what both mean to the total clinical picture. Some essentials of diagnostic reasoning are suggested, as is a handy reference outline for the complete physical exam.

Unit III, "Management Guidelines," is the heart of the book. Twelve chapters provide a condensed approach to disease management. This handy reference allows you to quickly locate the important information you need to diagnose and treat your patients effectively. Unit III begins with a discussion of common presenting symptoms seen in the primary-care setting, including an overview of differential diagnosis and diagnostically oriented algorithms to guide you toward the appropriate diagnosis and plan. Subsequent chapters include an assessment of each body system, followed by common disorders of that body system organized in a head-to-toe approach. The final chapter covers very important psychosocial problems, problems that nurses know can significantly affects one's health.

The discussion of each problem and disorder follows a consistent, easy-to-follow monograph format:

- Defintion
- Etiology
- Occurrence
- Age
- Ethnicity
- Gender
- Contributing Factors
- Signs and Symptoms
- Diagnostic tests
- Differential diagnosis
- Treatment
- Follow-up
- Sequelae
- Prevention/prophylaxis
- Referral
- Education

Educational resources, as well as ICD-9-CMs, are included. Unique features include specially designed flowcharts (algorithms) designed to assist the reader with decision making and treatment, as well as various tables, charts, and illustrations that condense important information.

Six very useful appendices are included: medication tables on commonly prescribed antibiotics, commonly prescribed nonsteroidal anti-inflammatory drugs (NSAIDs), prescribing topical steroids, commonly prescribed opioids, and an equianalgesic chart. Also included is an appendix containing the national telephone numbers of commonly used resources and services.

This book is written by—and for—advanced practice nurses involved in the day-to-day primary health care of adult patients. It provides you with the essentials of medical management required for safe and effective practice. However, it is your unique nursing-based perspective that differentiates and strengthens your application of these generic guidelines. Use this book and make it your own by jotting down experiences from your individual practice as well as new and updated medical treatment in the appropriate problem or discussion monograph. This will enable you to skillfully and knowledgeably bring to today's health-care arena things that we know our patients, today's health care consumers, are calling out for: astute, individualized, current, state-of-the-art, compassionate management of symptoms; an increased focus on quality of life and prevention; and perhaps most importantly, and simply, someone who listens to them, someone who cares for them, someone who hears them. This is what we, as advanced practice nurses, do best.

Lynne M. Hektor Dunphy

ACKNOWLEDGMENTS

Special acknowledgments to Roger A. Levy, MD, Diplomate of the American Board of Family Practice and Fellow, American Academy of Family Physicians, for his thoughtful medical review; and Pamela Lester, MSN, RN, ARNP, Family Nurse Practitioner, Western Communities Family Practice, Weelington, Florida, for her wise nursing review.

Additionally, a special thanks to Mary Jane Hopkins, MSN, RN, FNP, for her assistance in the development of the flowcharts.

L.M.H.D.

CONTRIBUTORS

Kim Bahnsen, BSN, RN-C, CCRN,
  CEN
ANP Student
Florida Atlantic University
Boca Raton, Florida
Educator
JFK Medical Center
Atlantis, Florida
  *Angina, Asthma, Congestive Heart
  Failure, Sleep Apnea, Upper
  Respiratory Infection*

Therese A. Boyd, EdD, RN, ANP-C,
  GNP-C
Adult Nurse Practitioner
Florida International University
  Student Health Services
North Miami, Florida
  Constipation, Palpitations

Naomi Breiner, MSN, ANP-C
Private Practice
Miami, Florida
  *Bell's Palsy, Brain Cancer,
  Cerebrovascular Accident,
  Encephalitis, Meningitis, Multiple
  Sclerosis, Parkinson's Disease,
  Seizures, Transient Ischemic
  Attack*

Nancie Bruce, DNSc, RN, CCRN
Adjunct Faculty College of
  Nursing
Florida Atlantic University
Boca Raton, Florida
  *Anaphylaxis; Bites—Animal and
  Human; Bites and Stings;
  Burns—Sunburn, Contact
  Photodermatitis*

Myra Buttacavoli, MSN, RN, PNP
Nurse Practitioner, Adolescent
  Medicine
Miami Children's Hospital
Miami, Florida
  *Rocky Mountain Spotted Fever,
  Sjögren's Syndrome*

Judy Chanin, MSN, RN
Doctoral Student
Univeristy of Miami, School of
  Nursing
Coral Gables, Florida
  *Bladder Cancer, Nephrolithiasis,
  Renal Failure—Acute and
  Chronic, Urinary Tract Infection*

Estelle J. Davis-Hodnett, MSN, RN, ANP
Nurse Practitioner, Primary Care
  Clinic
Miami Veterans Administration
  Medical Center
Miami, Florida
  Anorexia Nervosa, Bulimia,
    Insomnia

Loureen Downs, MSN, RN, FNP
Nurse Practitioner
Family Care Center
DelRay Beach, Florida
  Jaundice, Tuberculosis

Susan L. Folden, PhD, RN, FNP-C
Associate Professor, College of
  Nursing
Barry University
Miami Shores, Florida
Clinical Nurse Specialist
West Palm Beach Veterans
  Administration Medical Center
West Palm Beach, Florida
  Bronchitis, Chronic Obstructive
    Pulmonary Disease

Edward Freeman, PhD, RN, ANP, CS
Professor, School of Nursing
Barry University
Miami Shores, Florida
  HIV Disease

Joan Freeman, MSN, RN, ARNP
Nurse Practitioner, Women's Health
Private Practice
Hollywood, Florida
Adjunct Faculty, College of Nursing
Florida Atlantic Univeristy
Boca Raton, Florida
  Pancreatitis; Thyroid Cancer;
    Thyroid Imbalance:
    Goiter—Hyperthyroidism,
    Hypothyroidism

Terri L. Frock, EdD, RN
Assistant Professor, College of
  Nursing
Florida International University
North Miami, Florida
  Gastritis, Hepatitis

Julia Lynn Gamble, MSN, RN, FNP-C
Private Practice
Boca Raton, Florida
  Fibromyalgia, Infectious
    Mononucleosis

Lisa J. Granville, MD
Director, Acute Geriatric Unit
Miami Veterans Administration
  Medical Center
Miami, Florida
Assistant Professor of Clinical
  Medicine
University of Miami, School of
  Medicine
  Benign Prostatic Hyperplasia,
    Chancroid, Epididymitis, Erectile
    Dysfunction, Gonorrhea,
    Hoarseness, Human Papilloma
    Virus Infections, Hydrocele,
    Lymphogranuloma Venereum,
    Prostate Cancer, Prostatitis,
    Syphilis, Testicular Torsion,
    Urinary Incontinence, Varicocele

Elise Gropper, PhD, RN, CS
Faculty
Lynn University
Boca Raton, Florida
  Chapter 1—"Growth and
    Development: Health across the
    Life Span"

Kenneth W. Hazell, MSN, RN, FNP
Emergency Department
West Palm Beach Veterans
  Administration Medical Center
West Palm Beach, Florida
Adjunct Faculty/Doctoral Student
  (Nursing)
Barry University
Miami Shores, Florida
  Hearing Loss

**Linda J. Healy, MSN, RN, ANP,
CNS**
Nurse Practitioner, Cardiology
Private Practice
Miami, Florida
  *Mitral Valve Prolapse, Myocardial
  Infarction*

**Barbara Hegenmiller-Smith, MSN,
RN, ANP**
Nurse Practitioner
West Palm Beach Veterans
  Administration Medical Center
West Palm Beach, Florida
  Diabetes Mellitus—Types 1 and 2

**Lynne M. Hektor Dunphy, PhD,
RN, FNP, CS**
Associate Professor, College of
  Nursing
Florida Atlantic University
Boca Raton, Florida
Adjunct Nurse Researcher
Miami Veterans Administration
  Medical Center
Miami, Florida
  *Chapter 2—"Health Promotion,"
  Chapter 3—"Nutrition," Chapter
  13—"Musculoskeletal Disorders,"
  Chapter Assessment sections,
  Back Pain, Cough, Diarrhea,
  Dizziness, Glaucoma, Gout,
  Hernia, Hyperlipidemia, Lactose*

*Intolerance, Liver Cancer, Lyme
  Disease, Nausea and Vomiting,
  Oral Cancer, Panic Attack, Stasis
  Ulcer, Rheumatoid Arthritis,
  Osteoarthritis, Osteoporosis*

**Julie Hilsenbeck, MSN, RN, ANP,
CCRN, CNRN**
Director of Nursing Operations and
  Neuroscience Services
North Ridge Medical Services
North Ridge Medical Center
Fort Lauderdale, Florida
  *Bell's Palsy, Brain Cancer,
  Cerebrovascular Accident,
  Encephalitis, Meningitis, Multiple
  Sclerosis, Parkinson's Disease,
  Seizure Disorder, Transient
  Ischemic Attack*

**Mary Jane Hopkins, MSN, RN,
FNP-C**
Faculty, School of Nursing
Indian River Community College
Fort Pierce, Florida
  *Weight Loss, Fatigue,
  Gastroesophageal Reflux Disease,
  Obesity, Peptic Ulcer Disease,
  Syncope*

Ann Hubbard, MSN, RN, FNP-C
Faculty, School of Nursing
Indian River Community College
Fort Pierce, Florida
  Chest Pain, Costrochondritis

L. Renee Jester, MS, RN, FNP-C
Visiting Assistant Professor, College of
  Nursing
Florida Atlantic University
Boca Raton, Florida
  Fever

Joan Kelly, MSN, RN, FNP
Nurse Practitioner
Family Community Health Center
Okachobee, Florida
  Peripheral Vascular Disorders,
    Pneumonia, Raynaud's
    Phenomenon, Thrombophlebitis

Caryn King, MSN, RN, FNP-C
Private Practice
Delray Beach, Florida
  Colorectal Cancer, Pancreatic
    Cancer, Stomach Cancer,
    Thyroid Cancer

Janet M. Lakomy, PhD, RN, ANP
Adjunct Associate Professor, College
  of Nursing
Florida, Atlantic University
Boca Raton, Florida
  Cardiac Arrhythmias, Valvular
    Heart Disease

Susan Leacock, MSN, RN, ARNP
Acute Care Residency
  Program/Family Medicine
Jackson Memorial Hospital
Miami, Florida
  Acne, Burns, Cellulitis, Contact
    Dermatitis, Corns and Calluses,
    Ezcema, Herpes Zoster,
    Onychomycosis, Pediculosis,
    Psoriasis, Scabies, Seborrheic
    Dermatitis, Skin Cancer, Tinea,
    Uriticaria, Warts, Wounds

Nancy Leake, MSN, FNP-CS
Family Practice
Hollywood, Florida
  Cholecystitis, Cholelithiasis,
    Inflammatory Bowel Disease,
    Irritable Bowel Syndrome

Donna C. Maheady, EdD, RN,
  PNP-C
Visiting Assistant Professor, College of
  Nursing
Florida Atlantic University
Boca Raton, Florida
  Anal Fissure, Hemorrhoids

Janet E. Martin, MSN, RN, FNP-C
Adjunct Faculty, College of Nursing
Florida Atlantic University
Boca Raton, Florida
  Headache

Joanne Masella, MSN, RN, ANP-C
Faculty, School of Nursing
Palm Beach Community College
West Palm Beach, Florida
  Pleurisy

Ruth McCaffery, MSN, RN, FNP-C
Private Practice
Delray Beach, Florida
  Chronic Fatigue Syndrome

Marilyn Miller, PhD, RN, ANP-C
Assistant Professor, School of Nursing
Clemson University
Clemson, South Carolina
  Chapter 4—"History Taking,"
    Chapter 5—"Physical
    Examination and Clinical
    Decision Making"

Maura Miller, PhD, RN, GNP
Nurse Practioner, Long Term Care
West Palm Beach Veterans
  Administration Medical Center
West Palm Beach, Florida
  Pruritis

Rita Napier, MSN, RN, ANP-C, FNP-C
Adult Nurse Practitioner, Internal Medicine
West Palm Beach Veterans Administration Medical Center
West Palm Beach, Florida
Chalazion, Conjunctivitis, Hordeolum, Iritis, Peripheral Edema

Gilbert Nelmes, BS, PA
Private Practice, Orthopedics
Oxon Hill, Maryland
Bursitis, Carpal Tunnel Syndrome, Meniscal Tear, Sprains and Strains, Tendinitis

Edith F. Ortiz, MSN, RN, ANP
Nurse Practitioner, Psychiatry
Miami Veterans Administration Medical Center
Miami, Florida
Posttraumatic Stress Disorder

Aldona E. Paukstelis, MSN, RN, FNP-C
Senior Community Health Nurse
Health Department, State of Florida
Delray Beach, Florida
Gastroenteritis

Terri Pinder, MSN, RN, FNP
Staff Development Coordinator
Columbia Lawnwood Regional Medical Center
Fort Pierce, Florida
Epistaxis, Otitis Externa, Otitis Media

Brian Oscar Proter, BS, MD/PhD(c)
Researcher, Undergraduate Teaching Assistant
Department of Microbiology and Immunology
University of Miami School of Medicine
Miami, Florida
Candidiasis, Epistaxis, Herpes Simplex, Ménière's Disease, Otitis Externa, Otitis Media, Pharyngitis and Tonsillitis, Rhinitis, Sinusitis, Stomatitis, Temporal Arteritis

Janet Richards-Forbes, MSN, RN, ANP
Psychiatry
Miami Veterans Administration Medial Center
Miami, Florida
Abuse—Alcohol and Substance

Terry Rudes
Administrative Assistant
School of Nursing
Florida International University
Miami, Florida
Chapter 3—"Nutrition"

Lisa Silbert, MSN, RN, ANP, CNS, CCRN
Neurosurgical Nurse Practioner
Miami Veterans Administration Medical Center
Miami, Florida
Benign Prostatic Hyperplasia, Chancroid, Epididymitis, Erectile Dysfunction, Gonorrhea, Human Papilloma Virus Infections, Hydrocele, Lymphogranuloma Venereum, Prostate Cancer, Prostatitis, Syphilis, Testicular Torsion, Varicocele

Mary Healy Smith, MSN, RN, ANP
Nurse Practitioner/Research
    Coordinator Hypertension Clinic
Miami Veterans Administration
    Medical Center
Miami, Florida
Adjunct Faculty, College of Nursing
Florida International University
Miami, Florida
    Hypertension

Veronica P. Smith, BSN, RN
Coordinator, Substance
    Abuse/Posttraumatic Stress
    Disorder Program
Miami Veterans Administration
    Medical Center
Miami, Florida
    Depression

Gail Studer, MSN, RN, ANP
Nurse Practitioner
Private Practice
Boca Raton, Florida
    Appendicitis, Cirrhosis

Anne Thurston, MSN, RN, ANP
Nurse Practitioner
Private Practice
Silva, North Carolina
    *Acne, Burns, Cellulitis, Contact
    Dermatitis, Corns and Calluses,
    Eczema, Herpes Zoster,
    Onchomycosis, Pediculosis,
    Psoriasis, Scabies, Seborrheic
    Dermatitis, Skin Cancer, Tinea,
    Warts, Wounds*

Laura M. Villafane, BSN, RN
Nurse Liaison, Psychiatry
Miami Veterans Administration
    Medical Center
Miami, Florida
    Domestic Violence

Jill Winland-Brown, EdD, RN,
    FNP-C
Associate Professor, College of
    Nursing
Florida Atlantic University
Boca Raton, Florida
Nurse Practitioner
Private Practice
Boca Raton, Florida
    Anemias

REVIEWERS

Christine A. Boodley, RN, PhD
Associate Professor
University of Texas Medical Branch
School of Nursing
Galveston, Texas

Nancy Campbell-Heider, RN, PhD
Associate Professor
State University of New York at Buffalo
Buffalo, New York

Elizabeth Cohn, RN, MS, NP
Director of Clinical Research, Department of Cardiothoracic Surgery
Clinical Nurse III, Department of Emergency Medicine
North Shore University Hospital
Manhasset, New York

Mary Carol Galichia Pomatto, RN, MSN, EdD
Professor
Department of Nursing
Pittsburg State University
Pittsburg, Kansas

Denise Robinson, RN, PhD, FNP
Director, FNP Program and
    Family Nurse Practitioner, Student Health Center
Northern Kentucky University
Highland Heights, Kentucky
Family Nurse Practitioner
Northern Kentucky Family Health Centers, Inc.
Covington, Kentucky

CONTENTS

UNIT III
MANAGEMENT GUIDELINES